The "No Diet" Fat Loss Blueprint

Mark Broadbent

DISCLAIMER

This book, titled "The "No-Diet" Fat Loss Blueprint", is intended for informational purposes only and does not constitute professional medical advice, diagnosis, treatment, or recommendations of any kind. The reader should always consult their healthcare provider to determine the appropriateness of the information for their own situation or if they have any questions regarding a medical condition or treatment plan. Reading this book does not create a physician-patient relationship.

The author and publisher of this book have made every effort to ensure that the information provided herein is accurate and in accordance with the standards accepted at the time of publication. However, because scientific, medical, and health advice and guidelines continually evolve, the reader is urged to consult with a qualified healthcare provider for the most current information. No responsibility is assumed by the author or the publisher for any injury and/or damage to persons or property as a matter of products liability, negligence, or otherwise, or from any use or operation of any methods, products, instructions, or ideas contained in the material herein.

The recommendations, strategies, and tips described in this book may not be suitable for every individual and are not guaranteed or warranted to produce any particular results. Neither the publisher nor the author shall be liable for any physical, psychological, emotional, financial, or commercial damages, including, but not limited to, special, incidental, consequential, or other damages. The views and nutritional advice expressed are not intended to be a substitute for conventional medical service.

This book may contain references to other resources (books, articles, websites, etc.). These references are provided for informational purposes only and do not constitute an endorsement of any websites or other sources. Readers should be aware that the websites listed in this book may change.

WELCOME!

Congratulations on simplifying your nutrition!

I've been a Personal Trainer for over 20 years and I've seen all of the "Diets" going. Some stick around, some come and go, but most have one thing in common – they're difficult to stick to for most people because they tell you what you can or can't eat, and as soon as we're told we can't eat something… that's what we want to eat!

Not to mention it sucks the joy out of eating (and life!) when you want a burger, but order a salad, or when you have to count, weigh or measure every single thing you eat and drink every day!

Yes, your goal should be to gradually improve the way you eat, swapping "less healthy" options for "more healthy" options. Each and every step in the right direction takes you one step closer to your goals, but before we start restricting foods or force-feeding ourselves leaves, there are a number of things we can do.

These are your nutrition *habits*.

These habits are what differentiate the people who seem to be able to eat anything they want and stay slim, from those who just look at a cake and gain weight (no, I don't believe it's genetics, I believe the habits we pick up from our parents dictate our eating habits far more than the genes they gave us - our DNA hasn't changed in thousands of years, our habits and lifestyles have).

We can't get around the fact that calories do count, and "calories in vs calories out" is something we need to bear in mind, though it's not quite as simple as that because not all calories are equal, and the way your body responds to them varies (2,000 calories a day from chocolate bars will NOT yield the same result as 2,000 calories a day from quality meals, not just in terms of health, but also hunger, hormones, satiety, energy levels, health and happiness!).

This is why the calorie-counting method (or points, sins, red/green lights etc.) often fails people - because it's misleading, telling you to simply "stay within your calorie target and you'll be fine".

When these "Diets" fail, the Dieter often feels like a failure and is left frustrated and confused as to why "it works for other people" but not for them. What are they doing wrong?!

The No-Diet Fat Loss Blueprint will address your nutrition habits first. This is what dictates what, when and how you eat. If you can change your eating habits, you change what you eat by default. No stressing over what to eat (though it is better to consider things a little still), no need to go hungry (although when done properly, hunger isn't a bad thing as you'll see in lesson 7).

Habits are more permanent, more consistent and easier to follow than strict "Diets". We look to introduce them gradually, one step at a time, starting from where you feel comfortable right now, and then progressing as you feel able.

Yes, it can be a slightly longer process than a "90-day shred", but it'll be something you can stick with for the rest of your life – well beyond just 90 days of hell.

So, go through this book and introduce each habit as and when you feel able.

There's no need to do ALL of them right away, though there's no reason you couldn't.

Some habits you may find you naturally do already (whether

intentionally or not) and that's great! One less thing to think about!

I'll explain in each lesson ways you could start to introduce them. Most you can adjust up or down to your current level and then just look to build up gradually over time.

The key with habits is that they need to be so easy you don't have to think about it. It is exactly what is says on the tin – a "habit". Something you do automatically, without thinking about it.

You should be 90% confident that you can stick to the habit otherwise you'll need to dial it back a bit to a level you do feel at least 90% confident with. In a couple of weeks, it should start to become automatic and then you can look to move it forward a bit.

A little effort is required to begin with as you introduce a new habit, but given time and repetition, and if the habit is easy enough for you to follow right now, it'll soon become the automatic "habit" we want it to be.

In time, you'll be able to fine-tune all of these habits and stack them on top of each other.

Change just one thing for the better and it's a step in the right direction.

Change 2 or 3 things and it compounds – the sum is greater than the parts.

Soon enough your diet will likely be quite different to what it is now, and with almost no effort or hardship at all! And *a successful diet is one that you can stick to, <u>for good</u>*.

This is the key to long-term success with nutrition, and once you've mastered these habits, you can still go on to tweak things with regards to calories, food choices, adding in other habits and further improving on the ones you already do.

You may also be surprised to find that not all of the habits seem food related. Again, this is something most "Diets" fail to incorporate.

Good nutrition for *health* and fat loss is about much, much more than just what you do or don't eat. So, bear with me. Even if you can't see how one of these habits could aid in fat loss, it will contribute to your overall health, and a healthy body does not want to hold on to excess body fat.

Trust the process.

Eat Less and *Move More* are just two pieces of a much larger puzzle that we'll start to address in this book.

So...

Without further ado, let's jump in and start by busting a few myths around fat loss and dieting, then we can get into introducing your new habits :)

One more thing...

These habits, whilst complimentary, do not rely on each other to work.

Trying to change too much all at once may become overwhelming, which will almost certainly lead to failure.

While you should be tailoring each habit to your own achievable level, it may be a wise move to work on just one or two habits at a time.

This is a <u>long-term</u>, lifelong approach to health and nutrition. There's no rush.

Pick a habit, work on it for a week or two, then once it has become a "habit" (i.e. something you just do, without having to think about it), you can then add in the next habit... or further improve on that first habit and take it up a level.

I'd recommend you read through all of the habits first, and then pick one or two that seem the most achievable to you to begin with, or the one(s) that you feel will have the biggest impact on your health (Hint: Sleep and Hydration are great starting points!).

Then re-read whatever habit(s) you've chosen and set your level to whatever you think is achievable for you right now and start working on them.

Again, THERE'S NO RUSH!

This book isn't going anywhere. Don't feel you have to do all of this right away. The more pressure you feel, the more overwhelm, the less likely you are to even try it, let alone follow it.

Take it at a pace that's right for you.

Over time, you'll work on all of these habits and start to stack them on top of each other.

When you're "done" - *keep going.* Keep practising the habits you're doing and revisit each of them to see if you can further improve on it.

There's no end to this - we can always strive to make ourselves that little bit better.

Let's start by busting a few myths around Nutrition and fat loss...

MYTH #1

Thinking a "Diet" is something you do for X amount of time

There is no end date to good nutrition!

You'll probably have noticed already that I use the term "Diet" with a capital "D" and in inverted commas.

That's because a "Diet" is "thing" you "do" for a certain amount of time, before coming off of that "Diet". It's most likely the type of "Diet" that you're used to and have maybe "done" in the past.

In contrast, *your diet* is just something you do. No end date, it's not short-term, it's just the way you eat, and it will change as you do. It's flexible and lets you enjoy your food rather than stress about it, or worse, miss and crave food.

Your diet is everything you eat and drink, not a specific weight loss strategy.

Whilst many of these "Diets" work (because they all come down to the same basic principles), they tend to be strict, hard to stick to, and short term (predominantly *because* they're so hard to stick to).

Think about it – it's relatively easy to "follow a Diet" for a couple of weeks. A bit of hardship and going without… But imagine trying to eat like that forever… Not fun!

If you've ever followed one of these "Diets", you'll know exactly what I mean. It's the reason you're reading this book and not still following that "Diet!".

The <u>only</u> diet that works is the one you can stick to.

I'll repeat that:

The <u>only</u> diet that works is the one you can stick to.

Following a "Diet" and losing 10lbs *isn't* success if you then "come off" the "Diet" and gain that 10lbs back again.

That's a failed "Diet". It *didn't* work.

Whilst you may have a goal and a timeframe in which you'd *like* to achieve it (a holiday, a wedding, a work do…), it can be unhealthy to think of things in these terms. You really need to think long-term.

You should have the flexibility in your diet to tighten things up a bit for a week or two when you want to, but also enough control over what you eat and drink that maybe you don't actually need to.

By following a healthy diet, you'll naturally lose excess body fat because a healthy body doesn't want to carry around extra fat.

It's just a case of choosing the better options as often as possible, and not overeating.

So, get it out of your head that a "Diet" is something that has an end to it.

If the nutrition plan you're following makes you feel anxious about whether you could continue with it forever – *it's not going to work for you right now!*

You shouldn't have to "break your Diet" for a night out or a piece of birthday cake. Your diet should be flexible enough that you can accommodate those things and take them in your stride, without "ruining" things or "coming off the wagon".

So, I repeat, a good diet *has no end date.*

It doesn't cut out all the foods you enjoy.

It doesn't mean you have to either stay in or break your "Diet".

There's no such thing as a "cheat day".

There are no points, sins, coloured days or complicated recipes.

You don't have to eat specific meals at specific times.

And it shouldn't intimidate you.

Once you grasp some basic principles, like the ones in this book, you'll be able to go about your life without the stress of thinking about what you are or aren't "allowed" to eat.

Your weight will stabilise and you'll no longer swing from "Diet to lose a few lbs" to "put on a few lbs on holiday", to "Diet before Christmas", to "gain a few lbs over Christmas", to "Diet in January"… and on, and on…

So, let's move on, bust a couple more myths, and then get you back in control of your diet :)

MYTH #2

You have to be hungry when losing weight

You DO NOT have to go hungry in order to lose weight!

All successful weight loss diets (and "Diets") have a few things in common and one of them will always have to be a calorie deficit.

There's no escaping the fact that you have to burn more calories than you consume in order to lose weight, and have to consume more calories than you burn in order to gain weight.

BUT...

You absolutely don't have to be hungry when you're in a calorie deficit.

Most people instantly think of a "Diet" as going without the foods you love and being hungry all the time, and that doesn't have to be the case.

You may also have seen the "Diets" that advertise themselves by saying you can eat *more* and lose weight. These are actually on the right tracks, though still marketed to lure people in thinking they can just carry on as they are, even eat more and somehow lose weight.

This comes down to the fact that *all calories are NOT equal.*

There are some foods that have a large volume (very filling) with very few calories (Low Calorie Density) and will fill you up for very few calories.

There are other foods (normally the ones we like the most because they're designed that way) that have a lot of calories in a very small volume (High Calorie Density) – these are things like chocolate, cream, nuts and seeds, cheese etc. You can easily eat a huge number of calories from these without feeling full.

The key is to eat the High Calorie Density foods in moderation and fill up on the Low-Calorie Density foods.

This way you get to enjoy the foods you love still (sensibly) and never feel too hungry because you're still eating a lot of food.

This is how people came to be afraid of fats in the diet. Fats are high calorie density - meaning you can get a lot of calories from not a lot of fat - but this is a dangerous way of thinking and can often lead to people avoiding fats in the diet which leads to all manner of problems because [healthy] fats are *essential* in the diet and a great source of energy.

However, bear in mind that if your goal is fat loss, you need to be in a calorie deficit, and there's always a chance that you'll *want* more food than you can eat (especially if you're accustomed to overeating), but it's knowing the difference between being hungry (your body needing fuel) and simply *wanting* food that will help you control unnecessary eating.

In short, you don't have to be hungry to lose weight, but you will need to be in a calorie deficit, and the trick is to eat the right foods to avoid this. That said, hunger is a natural thing and shouldn't necessarily be avoided as you'll discover in habit 7.

MYTH #3

You can lose 10-years' worth of weight gain in a few weeks

Whilst it's possible to lose weight reasonably quickly, it's not healthy to do so, and often, the rebound of doing this leaves you right back where you started. Typical yo-yo Dieting.

It's likely taken you many years, a lifetime even, to get to where you are right now. People don't gain 100 lbs overnight; weight gain is a long process over many months and years.

The longer you've been overweight, the longer it's likely to take to regain your health.

This is another reason that a diet has to be sustainable - because you can't lose huge amounts of weight and reverse all health conditions in a few weeks, and you can't sustain a strict "Diet" for much more than a couple of weeks. Not to mention the fact that it would be unhealthy to do so (unless your current condition poses more of a threat to your health than the extreme Diet does).

I'm not saying that the gradual creep of weight over the last 1, 5, 10, 20 years will take as long to get off, but that you shouldn't expect miracles.

It's not just the weight gain that you're trying to reverse, it's also the 1, 5, 10, 20 years of eating habits that we need to address.

The faster you adopt these new healthy habits and make them a part of your life, the faster you'll see results, but years of bodily abuse will take its toll and can't be undone by eating salads for 2 weeks.

That said, you should start to see some results pretty quickly. A pound here, half a pound there…

To lose 10 stone you first have to lose 1lb, and that can happen pretty quickly.

Just remember that weight loss is not linear.

Some weeks you'll lose more than others.

Some weeks you'll lose nothing.

Some weeks you might even gain a pound or two again.

THIS IS NORMAL! And does <u>not</u> require you to keep changing what you're doing.

If the general trend of your weight is down, then you're doing the right things, keep going! As long as you don't gain weight for more than 2 or 3 weeks in a row, you're doing fine.

A general rule of thumb is that you can lose 0.5-1% of your bodyweight per week, but your focus, for long-term success, should be on <u>health</u> before weight loss, and changing your habits and your relationship with food is your priority, not the number on the scale right now.

Also, weight isn't the best measure of progress - it's *fat loss* most people are after, and we don't measure that on the scales, we measure it with bodyfat percentage and/or body measurements.

Don't be alarmed though, like I said, every step in the right direction helps so there's no reason that that first pound won't come right away, just don't get disheartened that 1lb isn't 2lb, or that 5lb isn't 10lb.

1lb at a time will get you there…

Fat loss is what we're after, not necessarily *weight* loss. There's a big difference.

A QUICK NOTE ON TRACKING BODYWEIGHT

Bodyweight doesn't tell us much. It's measuring bodyfat, yes, but also muscle tissue, bones, organs, stomach contents, hydration levels and more.

Any one of these can change your weight on the scales and it DOES NOT necessarily mean you're losing (or gaining) bodyfat.

IF you choose to track your weight, take daily measurements (first thing in the morning is best as the conditions are more consistent) and use the *weekly average* to compare week on week to see what progress you're making.

DO NOT start changing your diet or exercise routines because your "weight" changed by 1lb over night!

MYTH #4

Weight loss is just about eating less and moving more

We've addressed this already, "eat less, move more" is only true to an extent, because not all calories are equal, and under-eating and over-training will lead you to poor health instead of the good health we're aiming for.

Eating the *right* amount is better than simply eating less.

An *appropriate* exercise/training plan is better than just doing as much as you can.

Your aim should be to fuel your body with what it needs, no more, no less.

To gain, or at least maintain muscle mass whilst reducing stores of excess body fat.

To stress your body just enough for it to get stronger, not drain it to fatigue and leave you feeling worse instead of better.

Weight on the scales does not account for where that weight is coming from, so simply chasing a number on the scale doesn't guarantee success or health.

This is where a smart approach wins out every time. Rather than just focusing on weight on the scale, we look for other metrics to track, like body fat percentage, body measurements, progress photos, performance in your workouts, energy levels and how you *feel.*

Like the short term "Diets", excessive exercise can actually do the opposite of what it's supposed to and hinder your results.

Building healthy habits around both nutrition and exercise are what will get you the lasting results you're after, with far less effort than strict "Dieting" and burnout in the gym.

Yes, we aim to eat fewer calories (not necessarily less food) for fat loss.

Yes, we aim to incorporate exercise as an integral part of our health regime.

But simplifying it to just "eat less, move more" is misleading and has led a lot of people to frustration and failure.

We're about to change that for you now.

There are many more myths around fat loss, diet, exercise and health, but let's get into the meat of the course and start building your healthy habits.

See you in Habit 1!

HABIT 1 - SLOW DOWN

Ok, so here we are at the first habit!

Remember as you go through these that habits are built over time. You may be able to start some of these habits right now and stick to them for good, but chances are, to make them automatic, so you don't even have to think about them, it may take significantly longer.

I'd generally recommend practising each habit for a couple of weeks until it becomes almost automatic before introducing another new habit (or taking that habit to the next level), BUT... there's no reason why you wouldn't be able to start many or even all of these habits at the same time.

It may take a bit more brain power to begin with, as you have a number of things to remember and get used to, but if you're starting each habit at a level you're at least 90% (ideally 100%) confident that you can achieve and stick to, then it shouldn't be too much of a problem, and as I said before, the more healthy habits you can stack on top of each other, the better.

The more you do at once, the quicker you're likely to see and feel the results. That's why we look to continually improve on everything, forever!

Just be aware also, that if you try more than one thing at a time, it's hard to tell which of them is having the biggest impact, though this isn't really an issue because it doesn't matter too much as long as you're making progress.

So, Habit 1 – Slow Down

This is as simple as it sounds. Slow down when you eat.

Satiety hormones, hormones that tell your body *"I'm full, you can stop eating now"*, take a while to be released, and if you eat slowly, you'll recognise this signal (to stop eating) before you've overeaten.

If you eat quickly (especially calorie-dense foods), it's very easy to consume hundreds, even thousands more calories than you need long before the satiety signal is received by your brain.

Another good reason to slow down is for digestion.

Digestion starts in your mouth through chewing and saliva. You should be chewing your food thoroughly before you swallow it. This will make life far easier for your digestive system and reduce bloating and discomfort, and will help get more nutrients out of your food.

Thoroughly chewing your food will also take longer and naturally slow you down a bit.

There's a saying *"drink your food, chew your water"* which basically means you should chew your food to the point that it's basically liquid – completely pulverised and mixed with saliva; and chewing your water means you should swill it around your mouth a bit first, to mix it with the saliva, and also to get it to the right temperature before it hits your stomach (swallowing cold drinks isn't the best for your digestion).

Remember this as you eat, and it should slow you down a bit.

Another good tip is to put your knife and fork down between bites. Chew your food thoroughly and swallow it before you pick up your knife and fork to cut the next bite. Don't pre-load your fork with the next mouthful and have it waiting in your hand ready before you've even chewed the food in your mouth.

This will take some practice, but the act of slowing down can have a huge impact on both digestion and weight loss.

By slowing down and recognising when you're full, you could save yourself hundreds of calories a day, especially if you're not portioning out your meals appropriately (which most people are guilty of).

I'd advise that you don't rush meals. Sit down, take your time, and don't eat on the move.

Take a breath (or three) between mouthfuls, or a sip of water.

Savour and enjoy your food instead of getting it down you as quickly as possible.

There will always be times when you're in a rush but try to avoid these wherever possible by planning ahead and if you are eating quickly, make sure you've portioned out an appropriate amount of food or you'll just keep eating!

Don't get too distressed if this happens, as long as you're eating slowly and following the rule *most* of the time, the odd rushed meal won't ruin your efforts.

You may need to break old habits of eating quickly to master this habit, so it will take a conscious effort at every mealtime for a couple of weeks to really get the hang of it.

As simple as it sounds, this can actually be a tricky habit to take on. Have patience and stick with it. This one habit alone (as with all of these habits) could change your life!

HABIT 2 – STOP WHEN YOU'RE 80% FULL

Most people don't really know the difference between "full" and "stuffed".

They think that being full means you can't eat another bite and have to loosen your belt a notch.

This may have something to do with eating too quickly, as we addressed in the previous habit, but many of us were also raised to clear the plate.

IT'S NOT RUDE OR DISRESPECTFUL TO LEAVE SOME FOOD ON YOUR PLATE!

In fact, you may have experienced it when you finish your food only to be force-fed even more by your well-meaning Mum because they worry that they didn't give you enough! (my Mum is certainly like that, especially with the grandkids!!!). They mean well, but these 'feeders' only ingrain the habit of overeating in this situation.

Psychologically, you may feel you have to clear your plate because you've been conditioned to do so for whatever reason.

When you eat slowly, you'll start to recognise the difference between being full and overeating.

So, stop when you're 80% full. Even if you have food on your plate, stop.

Give it 5 or 10 minutes and I doubt you'll be thinking "I'm still hungry".

A trick I've told many, many people is to always (ALWAYS) leave a bite or two of food on your plate.

It breaks the mental block of having to clear the plate and teaches you it's ok to leave a bit.

We've all been there. Feeling stuffed but forcing down that one last bite just to finish our meal! *It's not ok!*

So, for the next two weeks at least, I challenge you to leave just one bite of food on your plate after <u>every</u> meal. Keep doing this until you've learned to recognise when you're full and aren't just eating to clear your plate.

Once you're able to recognise this and stop at 80% full, you don't have to leave one bite, you could leave more than that, or if your portions are right for you, you *might* clear the plate, but only because it's the right amount of food, not just for the sake of clearing your plate.

And if you do clear your plate, it doesn't mean you need more! No 'seconds!'

If you feel bad about wasting food – *get over it!*

This is more important right now, and it will teach you to dish up the correct portion sizes rather than just load up the plate. Get that right and you won't have to waste any food. You'll soon see that the amount of food you need is actually much less than you tend to pile on your plate.

HABIT 3 – DRINK MORE WATER

The vast majority of people nowadays walk around at some level of dehydration.

Very few of us actually drink adequate amounts of water, and even fewer still drink actual *water!*

Your body, as clever as it is, often mistakes thirst for hunger. So, if you're even slightly dehydrated, you may be thinking you're hungry when in fact you're just thirsty.

This is obviously a problem, because if you're chronically dehydrated you'll continually be looking for food because you think you're hungry.

There are many, many reasons why we need to stay hydrated, but from a weight loss perspective, staying fully hydrated can really help you to stop overeating.

Tea, coffee, fizzy drinks, alcohol, fruit juices don't really count. Yes, they'll get some fluids in you, but they bring problems of their own with regards to caffeine, sugar, calories, acidity levels etc.

Water is what we're supposed to drink. Plain old water.

So, Habit 3 is to **drink more water**.

How?

Drink 1-2 glasses of water upon waking (before your tea or coffee)

This will help to rehydrate you in the morning as we tend to get dehydrated overnight.

My tip is to take a bottle or pint of water up to bed with you and drink it as soon as you get up in the morning. Ideally include some electrolytes - either an electrolyte powder or a pinch of Celtic Sea Salt (see resources section for my recommendations).

If it's really a struggle to drink, you could add a Vitamin C tablet (check the ingredients and avoid aspartame where possible) or Berocca or similar to add some flavour and make it more palatable, but this shouldn't be necessary. If you really need to add some flavour you'd be better off squeezing half a lemon or lime into your water.

Drink a glass of water 10-15 minutes before *every* meal

This will prevent you mistaking thirst for hunger and can stop you from eating too much. It can also aid with digestion.

Sip on water throughout the day

A rule of thumb is to drink 1 litre of water for every 50lbs (about 22kg) of bodyweight, per day.

A couple of tips to do this are to carry a bottle of water around with you and make sure it's gone by the end of the day. You could even mark lines on the bottle so you know how much you should have drunk by 12pm, 3pm, 6pm etc...

Or set an alarm on your phone to remind you to drink every hour or two (there are even apps for this!).

Drink a glass of water any time you feel hungry or if you're looking for a snack

This, again, might just be thirst not hunger, so drinking a glass of water may actually stop you from having the snack, and will also keep you hydrated :)

Sip on electrolyte water during exercise and drink 2-3 glasses after exercise

This is to replace the fluids lost through sweating. Use an electrolyte powder or simply put some celtic sea salt in your water.

Increase your fluid intake on hot days or if you're on holiday somewhere hot

Again, to prevent dehydration, and including electrolytes is a good idea. Also, if you're particularly active, you'll likely need more water (even if you're not in a hot country or on holiday).

Front-load your water intake

It's better to drink a lot of water early in the day to rehydrate and ensure clear thinking and adequate hydration throughout the day. Also, if you fall behind, you don't want to be downing a litre of water before you go to bed! So, aim to drink at least half of your daily water by midday, then make sure to drink regularly after that using the tips above.

This protocol, if you're not used to drinking enough water, may leave you needing the toilet more than usual. This is logical (drink more, wee more), but also may be because your body isn't used to drinking this much water.

You will get more used to it, but adding the electrolytes to your water can help with this and it may stop you needing the toilet as often.

Remember though, it's more likely that you just didn't go to the toilet *enough* before because you were dehydrated, so going more now isn't a bad thing, it's helping your body flush out toxins and is essential for every cell in your body to function optimally.

If you don't like water...

Water is still the best thing we can drink, and I'd encourage you to try to drink water over tea/coffee etc wherever possible.

If you crave a bit of flavour, you could squeeze some lemon or lime juice into it.

You could try herbal/fruity teas, which you can also have cold in your water bottle throughout the day for a bit of flavour.

If you need some juice to add some flavour, just make sure you have it as weak as you can – you're trying to flavour your water, not drink pure sugar (or sweeteners!). Just get the least offensive one you can (i.e. no artificial colours, flavours or sweeteners and as few ingredients as possible) - adding a piece of fruit would be preferable to using squash or juice.

Try sparkling water – some people who don't like drinking still water do like sparkling water.

Add a vitamin C or multivitamin tablet to add flavour without using fruit juices or other things to sweeten your drinks (just check the ingredients - often they have a LOT more than just the vitamin C in them and are best avoided).

A note on water quality:

Where possible, avoid drinking tap water.

Bottled water is better, but there are still issues around the plastic bottles it's stored in.

If we're trying to improve our health and rehydrate, it's worth doing it properly, and if you're drinking multiple litres of water, every day, for the rest of your life - it's something worth investing in to make it as clean as possible. Even small traces of contaminants will build up over years of constant ingestion and can potentially cause major health issues further down the line.

My recommendation would be a Reverse Osmosis (R.O.) water filter (see resources for my recommendation).

It's the gold standard and relatively inexpensive.

Water is something you absolutely need and can't live without. You have to drink it every day. It's worth the investment to get a decent water filter so you can drink the best water possible.

The water filter jugs (you know the ones) simply don't cut it. They may be better than nothing, but in all honesty I think you should be aiming to get an R.O. water filter as soon as possible.

I'd also use, where possible, glass bottles rather than plastic (if you can find it in your local supermarket, grab a couple of bottles of Voss water – it may seem expensive for a bottle of water, but the bottle is worth it alone! You'd pay much more for a plastic water bottle with nothing in it!).

You could also use stainless steel or copper bottles, just avoid plastic!

HABIT 4 – USE A SMALLER PLATE

This could be one of the quickest, simplest tips ever – **use a smaller plate!**

If you're one of those people guilty of loading up your plate and have also been brought up to clear your plate, it could become quite obvious how any excess bodyfat could have accumulated over the years.

Unless you're following a recipe specifically for you and your calorie and macronutrient targets, chances are, your meals are just a bunch of ingredients thrown together with little thought given to the amounts.

Everyone's requirements are different so any recipe cannot possibly account for your personal calorie needs.

You then dish up what's been made, and that's what you eat; and if there's a little bit left (but not enough for another meal tomorrow), well… you finish it off so as not to waste it!

Well, it's very easy to overestimate how much food you actually need (especially when cooking things like rice, pasta, potatoes etc) and by filling a large plate with anything other than meat and vegetables, you're likely putting too much food on your plate.

The simplest solution to this is to use a smaller plate.

If you can't fit as much food on your plate, you won't be eating too much (and no, going back for "seconds" isn't allowed or it defeats the object!).

These meals may look small to begin with, but if you actually add up what's on your plate you'll probably find that it's about right for you if your goal is fat loss and you need a calorie deficit.

Prioritise protein (meat, fish, eggs etc.), then add your veg, and then, if your carbohydrate portion (pasta, rice, chips etc) looks a bit small - it's probably about right! It should fit in your cupped hand.

Failing that (if you, for some reason, feel a bit silly eating from a small plate), go for the posh restaurant look – a large plate with a lot of white space!

As a side note, it's a bugbear of mine when people feed their children adult-sized portions (particularly when those portions are too big for adults too!), so use the small plate for the kids too!

Yes, they're growing and need food, but overweight kids can really struggle with their weight later in life as they have a lifetime of poor eating habits to contend with!

Kids shouldn't be *too* skinny, but they definitely shouldn't be obese! We have an obesity epidemic in the western world and it's simply down to kids being overfed, particularly on poor quality, calorie-dense foods.

Just because they'll eat as much as you can put in front of them, doesn't mean you should keep feeding them! Swap that junk for some fresh vegetables and see how quickly they stop!

HABIT 5 – EAT PROTEIN AT EVERY MEAL

This is a big one.

It could have been habit 1, but really there's no order to these, you just adopt as many of these healthy habits as you can.

Protein is extremely important in our diet. It's your best friend when it comes to preserving or building muscle, and it fills you up for longer [than carbohydrates] as it takes longer to break down and digest; which is very helpful if you're trying to eat less!

When you train your muscles, you damage them a little bit so they grow back stronger ready to face that same stress again.

Your muscles need protein to do this, so a lack of protein in your diet will make it extremely difficult to build muscle tissue, or even maintain the muscle tissue you have.

Also, since fat loss is most peoples' aim, we want to tip the balance in favour of burning fat instead of burning muscle tissue – preserving muscle tissue through resistance training and eating plenty of protein is the number 1 way we can encourage our bodies to burn more fat for fuel and preserve valuable muscle tissue.

So, habit number 5 is this:

Make sure you eat protein at _every_ meal

The amount of protein we need varies depending on what literature you read, but 1.8-2.2g per kilogram of bodyweight (or roughly 1 gram per pound of bodyweight) is generally agreed to be the optimal range.

So, if you weigh 75kg (165 lbs) you'd be aiming to eat somewhere between 135-165g of protein per day.

This is a lot to eat in one or two sittings, so making sure you have protein at every meal will not only help to keep you feeling full up, it's the best way to ensure you're eating enough protein each day.

Most people tend to eat carbs for breakfast (cereal, toast etc.) and very little protein – **that needs to change**. It's very important to have protein at every meal. So, eggs and bacon are in. Chicken is in. Steak is in! YES!

Protein shakes are an option if you struggle to eat enough protein or if you "don't have time" to eat a proper breakfast. Real food is better, but if the option is a bowl of cereal or a protein shake – go for the shake.

To be clear, here are some examples of protein sources:

Meat
Fish
Eggs
Dairy
Protein supplements

Vegetarian options such as:

Tofu, Tempeh, Soy, Seitan, vegetarian/vegan protein supplements...

But these [vegetarian options] aren't as high in protein and don't tend to have all of the amino acids we need, so unless you're vegetarian for religious or ethical reasons, I'd strongly recommend you try to get your protein from the animal sources listed above.

A portion the size of your palm at each meal is a good starting point (think of a small to medium chicken breast, or a burger – about the same size and thickness as your hand).

The bigger you are, the bigger your hands will likely be, so the increased requirement for protein is covered beautifully using this simple method as your hands tend to be proportional to your body size.

If you're aiming to gain some muscle, you'll want to be aiming for the top end of the protein target and two palm-sized portions per meal may be more appropriate.

Also, if you're only eating a couple of times per day you may need to shoot for two palms instead of one or you simply won't hit your protein target.

So, for <u>*every meal you eat*</u>, ask yourself: *where's the protein?*

If there is none (or very little) – add some in, even if it means reducing something else.

Make your snacks protein too to help top it up (though you may not even need snacks if you're eating a good amount of protein and healthy fats in your main meals).

Snack examples could be:

Boiled eggs, Cottage cheese, Mozzarella ball, Tin of sardines, Protein shake, Meat, Tuna.

If you're hitting your protein target you may very well find that you feel hungry a lot less, snack a lot less and don't eat as much in general.

HABIT 6 – EAT YOUR VEGETABLES BUT USE THEM WISELY

Whilst I believe the carnivore diet is the most natural and logical human diet, and that fruit and veg would have been rare and seasonal and would not have made up a huge proportion of our diets, I do feel that there *can be* some benefit to eating them.

Predominantly, they can help fill you up and prevent you from overeating, and they're definitely less harmful than the usual junk food people eat and fill up on.

Fruit and veg are low calorie-density foods, meaning they don't carry a lot of calories for their weight/size. If you've ever seen/heard people saying you can "eat more and lose weight" - this is what they're referring to. You can eat a huge volume of food for relatively few calories.

Whilst I don't recommend stuffing yourself with as much veg as you can, it does mean you can use them to help you feel full and prevent snacking.

You can also get some fibre and micronutrients from them which you may struggle to get purely from meat unless you're regularly eating organ meats too.

I'd always recommend trying to eat organic, local and seasonal veg, and limit it so you're not overdoing it.

If you follow the previous habit, you'll be ensuring you're getting your most vital nutrient, protein, and if you do that, you'll likely struggle to overeat anyway.

Ensure you've got enough protein on your plate, then, if you like or need to, add in the veg to fill it out a bit and fill you up - rather than loading up on starchy carbs like rice, pasta, chips etc.

Fruit is actually less of an insult to our bodies (it's the part of the plant that's actually supposed to be eaten, so it doesn't contain the same chemicals as plants [veg] do).

If you're eating the whole fruit (not just the juice), with its fibre, it's something your body can deal with.

Same rules apply though - try to get fresh, organic, local and seasonal fruit, and don't overdo it.

If you're going to overdo anything though, it's better that it be organic fruit than sweets and crisps!

Start by replacing the junk with something *better* and then you can taper that off too later on, if you need to.

Our ancestors would NOT have had access to fruit and vegetables year-round. It would have been small amounts at certain times of the year, so it seems illogical that they'd be essential for our health.

By all means top-up your diet with them, but don't overdo it.

HABIT 7 – HAVE AT LEAST A 12-HOUR BREAK FROM EATING EACH DAY

Intermittent Fasting has become a bit of a "thing" over the last few years. Everyone's heard of it and it seems big and scary and complicated.

In reality, giving it a name, "Intermittent Fasting", is what's caused the problem.

There should be zero controversy around fasting, and whilst, like diet, it *could* get very complex, it doesn't have to and is actually the simplest thing you can do.

We are designed for feast and famine.

Periods without food (because a hunt was unsuccessful and nothing's growing) followed by periods of feast (when a hunt goes well and you bring back 200lbs of wild animal!).

Our bodies have evolved with mechanisms to deal with this cycle and are well adapted for it. Straying from this pattern is *un-natural*.

Many things happen in our bodies when we are fasting and many of the health benefits of fasting start to kick in at around the 12-13 hour mark.

It's completely natural to go *at least* this amount of time without eating.

The difference between eating 2,000 calories within an 8-12 hour window, followed by a 12-16 hour fast, and eating 2,000 calories spread throughout the day, is that your body never gets a chance to rest if you're constantly eating.

Your digestive system never gets a chance to rest, and the hormones that are released and the protective mechanisms that kick in when you're fasting don't get a chance to do their work.

"Little and often" or "grazing" *ISN'T* natural.

Whilst the total daily calories are the same, the results from these two ways of eating are wildly different.

It needs to be remembered that fasting should be done for the _health benefits_, NOT for "weight loss" – and that's where it goes horribly wrong for many, and where any horror stories come from.

It can however work very well as an *aid* to weight loss :)

This is simply because, by adopting this Time Restricted Feeding protocol, you're setting yourself a cut-off time each day when you stop consuming any calories.

For a lot of people, it's quite common (habitual) to eat/drink anywhere from a couple of hundred calories to a couple of thousand calories after dinner, in front of the TV before bed.

By eliminating this needless snacking, you could realistically save yourself a few hundred calories a day – enough to see some weight loss without doing *anything* other than setting yourself a cut-off time for eating or drinking anything with calories in.

Your 12 hours starts from the moment you finish your last bite of food/sip of drink.

After that time, you eat nothing and drink only calorie-free drinks (not coke etc or "Diet" versions of stuff – just water or herbal/fruit teas).

You should try to make this cut-off time around 2-3 hours before bed so you're also not going to sleep with food still digesting in your stomach.

As far as dieting goes – it doesn't get any simpler.

"Stop eating by 8pm" (or whatever time you've chosen, working backwards from your bedtime).

The clock stops 12-13 hours later when you can have your first bite of food or calorie-containing drink - or "breakfast" (breaking the fast - whatever time of day that happens to be).

Stop eating at 7pm, have breakfast no sooner than 7am.

Stop eating at 9pm, have breakfast no sooner than 9am.

You get the idea.

Hunger doesn't just build and build so don't panic. Also, doing it like this, you'll be sleeping for most of this time and the first few hours are right after dinner, so you shouldn't be hungry then either.

The simplest way to think of this habit is just stop eating at X time and don't snack between dinner and bedtime. *That's it!*

If you have any medical conditions or need to take medications with food, I'd definitely recommend speaking to your doctor about this first and figuring out how you can work this around your medications.

As you get used to this, it may be worth experimenting with shortening your "eating window" and extending your fasting time.

The 16:8 protocol has a lot of merit and *could* be something to work towards if you feel you'd benefit from this.

People often succumb to hunger, but accepting hunger and accepting that it's a natural sensation that we're *supposed* to experience helps.

Also, if you pay attention, you'll notice that hunger doesn't just grow and grow, it comes and goes. You could feel starving at one moment, then be absolutely fine half an hour later.

It comes and goes in waves and you just have to get through it. Have a big glass of water and do something to keep busy.

You've got enough stored energy on your body to last you weeks, even months! You won't starve by being a bit hungry for an hour!

Avoiding hunger isn't necessary. Just accept it as something that happens.

HABIT 8 – SLEEP 7-9 HOURS EVERY NIGHT

Sleep is one of THE most important things you can do. It's when your body rests, repairs and grows and you CANNOT enjoy good health without it.

A lack of sleep impairs both physical and mental performance (a lot more than you'd believe!).

There's a reason why shift work has been classed as a possible carcinogen (cancer-causing).

If you want your body to recover from workouts, stressful days or illness, you'll need to get your sleep.

It'll also do more to keep you youthful (for FREE!) than any "anti-ageing" products that cost fortunes!

The best way to ensure you get enough sleep (of good quality too) is to have a regular bedtime and wake-up time (even at the weekends) so your body can set its daily rhythm.

This will help you to fall asleep and wake up more easily at the same times each day and will also improve sleep quality.

Be consistent with these.

Bedtime routine:

Turn off all screens and bright lights as early as you can (ideally at least an hour before bed) – use only dim lights (not bright LED's!). I like the Himalayan salt lamps (link in resources).

Do something relaxing – bath, reading, stretching, listen to some music, play a game, talk (not on the phone).

Sleep in pitch black – ensure your room is dark and cool. No lights whatsoever (even the LED on your TV or an alarm clock).

Leave your phone in another room – you DO NOT need it in your bedroom! If you use it as an alarm – ditch it and get an alarm clock, ideally a sunrise alarm clock (again, link in resources).

Try a herbal tea before bed – the "nighttime" teas have herbs in them that can help you relax.

Take some Magnesium half an hour before bed – it can help you relax and sleep better (follow the dosage on the packet). I like the magnesium spray. (You can find my recommended products at www.MoveBetter.Club/recommended)

Remember: weekends aren't for staying up late and getting up late. If you want to give yourself "jetlag" every Monday morning, this is exactly how to do it!

Routine is your friend.

Make this a habit you don't ignore.

Before you state that you're one of those people who "doesn't need that much sleep" – I disagree!

You may think that, but if you read into it, you'll learn that this accounts for approximately 0% of the population. We all need 7-9 hours, VERY few people can get away with less without some kind of impairment, even if you don't notice it.

In fact, driving tired is more dangerous than driving under the influence of alcohol (unless you're waaay over the limit at least). Driving tired causes more accidents than alcohol, not just at night, but any time of day if you haven't slept well.

Further reading on this is HIGHLY recommended – it's that important! Again, check out the resources section for my recommendations, but I also have another book called *"The Ultimate Sleep Solution"* available on amazon which I'd encourage you to check out - it has 17 simple steps you can follow to fix your poor sleep <u>without</u> pills or potions!

But for now, just set your bedtime and wake up time and stick to it, making sure you get at least 7 hours per night, but ideally 8 or 9.

You don't have to know the "why" to enjoy the benefits of doing this.

HABIT 9 – MOVE DAILY

There's no avoiding it, we're designed to move our bodies. A lot. Every day.

So, habit number 9 is to do just that. *Move.*

10,000 steps a day is your goal, but you can measure where you are right now and just aim to increase that a bit each week.

Like the other habits, it's not *all or nothing*, it's *do what you can now with a view to improving on that further in the future.*

If you're currently doing 5,000 steps a day consistently, make your goal to hit 7,000 steps a day.

When you can do that consistently, aim for 8,500 or 9,000.

Again, when you're doing that *consistently*, aim for 10,000.

Aim for *progress* not perfection (with all of these habits).

Some days will be higher than others, but we're looking for the <u>average</u> number of steps per day. Add them up and divide by 7 each week or aim for a weekly goal (10,000 steps a day is 70,000 steps a week; 5,000 a day is 35,000 a week…).

Use the checklist in the bonuses to check off each day that you hit your target. If you miss a day, try your best to make up the extra steps the following day.

Quick Tip:

Try to get above your step target as early in the week as you can – it'll give you a bit more flexibility later in the week if there are days you fall a bit under, or it will bump up your weekly total if you don't miss any days; but if you are under in the first couple of days, it gives you very little flexibility when it comes to making up those steps later in the week.

You could also aim to do this daily too - aim to get the bulk of your steps in early on to give a little more flexibility if things get busy during the day (it's too easy to get busy and then be nowhere near your steps by the end of the day!).

This is a good rule for life - **Do the important things <u>first</u>!**

I will mention that 10,000 steps a day, originally, came from a marketing campaign for pedometers back in the 60's and had very little, if any, scientific backing, *however* it **is** a reasonable and achievable number to aim for.

As a bare minimum I'd recommend that everyone should get *at least* 7,000 steps a day.

So that's "exercise"....

Now let's talk about *Training*.

Exercise is your daily movement. Training is your specified workout time with a specific goal in mind.

For most (even if fat loss is the goal) this means strength training – working your muscles to maintain or build them up, gain strength, and encourage your body to hold on to muscle tissue and burn fat tissue.

Dieting without resistance training can lead to you losing the wrong "weight". If Fat Loss is the goal, you want that weight to come from fat stores on the body, not from muscle tissue. By training with resistance you're signalling to your body to keep hold of (or even build) muscle tissue and break down fat stores.

A calorie deficit *without* resistance training tends to break down much more muscle tissue [relatively] and less fat tissue as compared to a calorie deficit paired with strength training.

Cardio isn't a complete waste of time, but your *training* time should focus on strength, and let your daily movement/exercise take care of the steps.

Unless you're specifically training for a marathon or some other "cardio" type event, then strength training should be your priority and you can add your "cardio" in outside of this.

It is still important to train "cardio" and I'm not saying don't, I'm saying *prioritise* strength training. Get that done first, then if you can, add in some dedicated cardio work (or you can do the old classic of adding it in for 20 minutes at the end of your workouts).

You can start small, just 10-20 minutes every other day will be fine. Then, again, build it up as you get more accustomed to it and as it becomes more of a habit.

You should ultimately aim to do strength training 3-4 times a week, for 30-60 minutes, increasing the intensity as you progress.

The details of strength training routines are too much to include in this book but I've included a general plan that covers most of the bases in the bonus/resources section, or you can also head to www.MoveBetter.Club where you can sign up and get access to dozens of workouts and multiple training plans written by me which are far better than any bodybuilding-style training plan you'll get off google.

And since my goal is to help you get as healthy as possible, we can't forget about mobility work – this should be incorporated into your strength training routines, but also into your daily life.

Yes, walking is good and we're aiming for 10,000 steps, but if you want to keep your body *moving well* long into the future, you need to keep it moving <u>now</u>.

I have a 5-Minute Mobility Routine that you can follow along with, again, in the resources section – that's a great start and if you do that once or twice a day it'll really help to keep your joints moving the way they should.

Remember though this is only a start, you may need something more focused to address any imbalances or tightness you have personally. If that's the case, or when you're ready to take things up a notch, it's worth hiring a Coach to help guide you and make sure you're doing the right things.

To summarise Habit 9…

9.1 Set your daily or weekly step targets and hit that target!

9.2 Go through a mobility routine (either full body or specific to you) 1-2 times daily

9.3 Strength train 3-4 times a week (again, you could start at 2x20 minute sessions, then build up as the weeks progress). Fill the rest of the time while you're building up with your "cardio" work.

By all means look at these as 3 separate habits and address them each individually. If you need to start with just one or two of them then do that and when they become "habit", not forced, you can add in the next one.

Maybe this will be another book, but for now, you can get multiple workouts and training plans on my membership site www.MoveBetter.Club - it's a great place to start (and possibly all you'll ever need).

Bonus #1
The "Thousand Recipe Code"

We've all bought a recipe book thinking we'll eat healthily from now on… Just follow the recipes – it's easy!

But let's face it, we've all got a dozen of those recipe books in a cupboard somewhere, not because we've memorised all of the recipes, but because the novelty wore off and it's easier to revert back to old ways because you've rarely got the ingredients necessary to cook half of the meals in there.

Sure, some of what you learned might have stuck, but for the most part, you're back where you started.

THIS bonus will help you create a healthy meal, simply, without the need to get the book out and find a recipe that you A) want, and B) actually have the ingredients for.

You can use this method to create literally thousands of different meals.

You'll probably lean towards a lot of the same ingredients – we all have things we like and eat often – but this will help you make each meal different, even if you're using the same base ingredients.

Chicken and rice will never be the same again! Hallelujah!

However, I do still recommend you try to vary your diet as much as possible. Rotate between various meats, vegetables, fats etc. It helps keep things interesting but will also ensure you're getting a variety of nutrients.

If you eat the same meat and the same veg *all* the time, you'll be missing out on any nutrients they may be lacking. The only way to ensure you're getting everything you need from your diet is to vary it and eat a wide variety of food.

Eat the rainbow. Try and get as many different colours on your plate as you can, or at least change the colour of each meal – different coloured vegetables contain different nutrients, so mix them up.

So... the magic code...

It's as simple as this:

- Choose your protein (because it's the basis of every meal remember)

Meat, organ meats, fish, eggs, dairy, vegetarian options...

- Choose your veg and/or fruit (1-3 different vegetables)

- Choose your carb source (potato, rice, bulgur wheat, quinoa, chickpeas etc)

- Choose a healthy fat (olive oil if cold, coconut oil, avocado oil, butter, avocado, nuts, seeds...)

Those are the basis of your meal – Protein, carb, healthy fat and veg.

Then...

Portion them appropriately using your hand as a guide:

1-2 palms for your protein

1-2 fists of veg

1-2 cupped hands of your carbs (fair warning: This will likely be much less than you're used to piling on your plate!)

1-2 thumbs of fats

(I understand that "1-2 palms" is a little vague, but this depends on your goals - fat loss or muscle gain - and how frequently you're eating - 2 meals a day? 3? 4?...)

If you're looking to gain weight, go for 2; to lose weight, go for one; to gain muscle - 2 for protein, one for carbs...

You get the idea, you'll need to figure out what works for you or get some extra guidance from a coach who knows what they're talking about (if they just give you a calorie target - move on!).

Next, choose your garnishes/flavours.

This is where you can get creative. Choose the herbs and spices you like, or pick a regional flavour to go for – Italian, Spanish, Turkish, French, Indian, Moroccan... Just use the traditional herbs and spices of those countries to add a twist to your meal.

3 or 4 (or more) of these will give you enough combinations to almost never repeat a meal! There are dozens of flavours to choose from, and literally thousands of combinations you could try.

Tip: Make a note of what you use when you make a meal, and if you like it, you can use it again. Likewise, if there's a flavour combination you're not so keen on, you'll know not to use it again.

As well as herbs and spices, you can also use butter, chillies, garlic, lemons and limes or sauces (preferably freshly prepared to avoid excessive added ingredients!).

Finally, cook the food!

Again, how you cook it can make a difference.

You could pan fry, grill, bake, stir-fry, BBQ, Air-Fry, slow cook or any other method you choose.

You really can make dozens of different meals from the same ingredients by using a few simple tweaks with flavours and cooking methods.

And when you're in a rush, you don't even need to think about it – chuck your meat in a pan, add the veg, throw in some flavours then serve with your chosen carb and drizzle with healthy fats. Voila!

This is essentially what many "Fitness Food" bars do – you select your protein, your carb and your veg, then choose which flavour sauce you'd like it with. A meal to suit any palate.

If your spice rack is lacking, buy some new flavours on your next trip to the supermarket. Pick the ones that appeal to you.

Get a good selection of herbs and spices, or as a backup (lazy option) some different sauces to flavour your food with.

You can't get this wrong!

Give it a try and see how you get on.

Bonus #2
A guide to restaurant eating

If you've "Dieted" before, you'll know the pain when it comes to eating out.

The menu doesn't have the calories on it, let alone the proteins, carbs and fats in each meal.

They're set to one size, so like a random recipe in a book, the portions won't be appropriate for everyone.

On top of that, you want dessert and a glass (or three) of wine or a beer with it.

"Diet" out the window!

But it doesn't have to be.

Firstly, remember that you're the boss, the customer, and you can ask for changes to the meal.

Want a steak but trying to reduce carbs? Ask for some veg instead of chips.

Want the burger but without the cheese? Just ask.

Trying to cut back on bread? Have the burger but leave the bun, or just have half of the bun.

Also remember, you don't *have* to clear your plate. Leave a bite or two. Leave a few chips. Leave some of the rice. It's fine!

Use your hand-size guide to gauge how much you should be eating and if there's too much on the plate, leave it.

Just because you've paid for that meal (as if you don't pay for the rest of your meals) doesn't mean you're wasting money if you don't finish it. A few bites left on the plate won't make a difference to your bank balance, but it could make a difference to your progress.

The best tip though is to plan ahead. Most of the time you will have to book your table, which means you *know* where you're eating.

Look at the menu in advance and choose what you're going to have (or at least narrow it down to a couple of options that are most in-keeping with your nutrition plan). If you can't access the menu beforehand, it could be worth eating somewhere else.

Everywhere sells steak – add some veg and you're spot on with your diet. If you keep it to just steak and veg, you've also got some carbs left over for dessert too.

Yes, you may go slightly over on 'calories' for that meal, but if you know that in advance you *could* (but don't have to) have a smaller lunch that day, or a smaller lunch the following day.

DON'T stuff your face and then starve yourself the next day, but you <u>can</u> eat a little extra and reduce calories slightly on the days around it to compensate.

As for drinks, there's no getting around it, they contain calories, sugars, and zero nutrition, but as I said, if you've limited your carbs in your meal, you can allocate some of those to your drinks.

You could also, as I mentioned before, reduce your carbs earlier on in the day knowing you're going to have a drink that night with your meal.

The main thing is to not get stressed over it, and definitely don't throw the diet out the window and have a blowout.

A drink because you enjoy it is one thing. Drinking to get drunk is pointless and will absolutely be detrimental to your progress, so think hard about what's more important – achieving your long-term goals, or a drunken night followed by guilt, regret, and feeling like crap?!

You can easily drink through an entire week's worth of calorie deficit in one night – don't undo all your hard work every weekend or you'll get nowhere.

Eating out doesn't have to mean ruining your hard work and can actually be beneficial to your diet, because we're not supposed to eat the exact same number of calories day in, day out.

Fluctuations do and must happen, so a slightly lower calorie day alternated with a slightly higher calorie day (which balance out to your daily calorie target) are actually extremely beneficial and will keep your body from adapting to a reduced calorie intake and slowing down the fat burning process. People also often eat things they wouldn't normally have when eating out, so it can add a bit of variety to your diet too.

I hate the terms "cheat meal" or "cheat day" as they imply you can eat what you want with no consequence and have to be 'strict' for the rest of the week, but a pre-planned refeed where you eat a few more calories than your daily target (from the same good foods still) is a good thing every now and then (the more weight you want to lose, the less frequent these should be, but as you get nearer and nearer your goal weight/bodyfat percentage, you can increase the frequency of these refeeds accordingly).

It's better to fluctuate your calories daily for a weekly total than to have the exact same target 7 days a week anyway.

A much better way to think of it though is to just alternate between the higher and lower intake days.

I must stress though, that whilst you can plan for a slightly higher calorie intake and even increase your activity levels in the days surrounding this, DO NOT use exercise as a "punishment" for over-eating, and equally don't use the fact you've done your exercise as an excuse to eat more 9two things I've seen a lot over the years!).

DO NOT reward your hard work with exercise and nutrition with food and drink - choose rewards that are more appropriate.

Too many people work so hard following a nutrition and exercise plan and then go on to 'reward' themselves with the very things they've been trying to limit - this is a telltale sign that the "Diet" they've been following isn't sustainable and won't yield results long-term.

If the fact that you're healthier, and look and feel better aren't reward enough, then by all means reward your efforts with something else, but don't use food. Book yourself a massage or buy that top you wanted now you're a size smaller. Pick something that's in-keeping with your new, healthier lifestyle.

A final tip, when it comes to choosing your meal, just go for the "healthier" option. It doesn't have to be a salad, but if your options are a large pizza or a medium pizza – go for the medium and mitigate the damage.

Instead of a greasy doner kebab, have the shish.

A burger would be better than a pizza.

Grilled chicken would be better than fried chicken.

You get the idea, if you can just choose the *healthier* option, the "less bad" option, you'll always save yourself a few calories.

Eating out does not mean a diet ruined. Enjoy yourself sensibly and keep in mind what you're trying to achieve.

One last note on drinks - whilst you *can* choose 'diet' or 'zero-calorie' drinks, the sugars they've taken out are replaced with other chemical sweeteners, so while it may save you some calories, the health implications of consuming these additives and chemicals are, for me at least, just not worth it, and not what this book is about.

Also, regardless of calorie content, alcohol just isn't good for us and will only damage your health. Sorry.

CONSISTENCY IS KEY

You won't get it right 100% of the time.

Aim for progress not perfection.

It's easy to start some things and then let them taper off until you've forgotten you even did it to begin with.

The true key to success isn't how hard you work (well, that does come into it) but how <u>consistent</u> you are with the things you choose to do.

Consistency beats intensity every time.

Use the daily habit checklist in the resources section to help you stay consistent.

No-one is expecting you to be perfect, I'm certainly not, and neither should you.

Following something 100% for a few weeks is great, but if that's unsustainable it'll soon stop and you'll be right back where you started.

That's why these habits are so simple and so powerful. They can all be adapted to your current level or ability, and tweaked as you go.

By adapting each habit to your current level, you should be able to follow them at least 80% of the time and that's what we're aiming for.

100% is great and totally achievable if you have the habit set to your level, but don't panic if you don't manage 100% - we all have the odd late night, a few too many, or an extra slice of cake. That's life, it's for enjoying, and you should let yourself do the things you want... within reason.

If you're struggling with any of the habits, review it.

Ask yourself WHY you're struggling. What specifically are you struggling with?

Dial back on the habit a bit and start there.

As an example, if you're aiming to have 4 workouts per week, but only managing 3, then ask yourself if 4 is realistic right now.

Could you do the three then make the fourth a short, 20-minute home workout?

Could you get up half an hour earlier one day to squeeze the 4th workout in?

Or is 4 just completely unrealistic for you right now?

Answer these questions and either find a solution, or adjust your expectations accordingly.

Three workouts might be enough anyway, but if it's not, just adjust your time-frame and build up to it. Get used to the 3, then figure out how you can fit the 4th in when you're ready - it may mean sacrificing something else but weigh up your priorities and make the decision. Do or don't.

These habits have to become just that - *habits.*
Not something you have to think about.

It'll take time. Some habits may only take a couple of weeks to establish, others may take months, even years! Persevere with them and you'll enjoy the benefits for the rest of your life.

When you *automatically* choose the healthiest menu option, or just get up and put on your gym kit, or drink water constantly throughout the day without needing a reminder - *that's a habit.*

When these habits become *'habits'*, you will be consistent with no effort at all.

I'd rather you ate 5 pieces of veg a day, drank 2 litres of water a day, and trained twice a week, *forever*, than ate 10 pieces of veg, trained 6 days a week and drank 4 litres of water for 3 weeks and then stopped.

Your goal is consistency.

Be consistent.

You got this!

It's also worth saying though that if a habit seems too easy, you may need to adjust it UP a bit. Challenge yourself a little to fast-track the results.

For example, if drinking 1 litre of water a day is so easy you don't have to think about it - that's a habit; but we want to push this a bit more. Maybe increase your target to 2 litres, so you have to think about it a little more, but it's achievable with a little effort.

Obviously for some habits there's a limit (i.e. you don't want to continually add more and more water beyond your target, and the same with protein etc.) so once you reach your goal - that's fantastic! Keep it going and focus your attention on another habit.

Make it right FOR YOU.

Add new habits or improve on old ones as and when you're ready.

It's an ongoing process that will never end and there's no limit to how much you can improve and get out of it, so always keep working on yourself

YOUR DAILY CHECKLIST

If you don't track it, you can't measure it.

Often people think they're doing something when they're not (make a food diary and compare it to what you *think* you eat - I guarantee you'll see stuff on there you didn't remember eating! Under-reporting is so common on a food diary it's almost funny!).

The point is - *track your progress.*

I've added a checklist in the resources section that you can print out and put on the fridge (or carry around with you) and tick off each day that you complete that habit. By all means add some of your own, just remember not to try and do too much all at once - maybe add new habits one by one once you've mastered these first ones.

At the end of the week/month/year you can look back on this and see how you're doing.

Also track anything you'd like to keep an eye on - workout performance, recovery, HRV, RHR, bodyfat percentage, weight, body measurements, progress photos, energy levels, sleep, blood pressure, hair/skin/nail condition, how you feel, mood...

Anything you want to change needs to be tracked (or else how will you know if what you're doing is working or not?!). Just pick the appropriate metrics to track based on your goals.

Just remember - weighing yourself every day won't change your weight - your habits will. So once you've set your goals and know what metrics you want to change and track, you need to establish what *habits/actions/behaviours* you need to adopt to move you towards those goals, then use your daily habits checklist to ensure you're *doing* what you need to do to get the results you want to achieve.

If you're not regularly ticking off the required actions/behaviours, you'll know why your results are the way they are.

You'll be surprised how much difference the habits in this book can make once you incorporate them consistently and it should show on your tracking sheet.

Print out the checklist and fill in what's relevant for you, then tick it off as you go.

As you master each habit, you can increase it slightly up to your desired end point (i.e. you may be starting at 7 hours of sleep per night with the goal to eventually get it up to 9 hours).

Troubleshooting Problems you could expect to encounter and what to do about them

This section could easily take up an entire book because everyone struggles with different things. It all depends on your current/ past habits and how easy you'll find it to change them or incorporate new, healthier habits into your routine.

Each habit can come with its own problems, but if you use the advice given and scale all habits down to a level you're at least 90% confident you can do, then you should be alright.

I've tried to give tips on each of the habits to ensure you don't encounter any problems, but here are a couple of things you may be a bit unsure of.

Work shifts and can't get a regular sleep/wake schedule going on?

Don't panic. Control what you can. Get a routine together for the days you work in the day, and a separate routine for when you work nights - the main focus here would be to get as much light as you can in the day, and dim the lights a couple of hours before bed and sleep in the pitch black. Set up your bedtime routine and do it before bed each day.

13 hours seems like a long time to go without food?

Start at 11 or 12, just aim to build it up to 13 or 14 in a few weeks' time. Hunger comes and goes, it doesn't build. It's often a psychological barrier, not physiological, so once you realise it's actually not that bad, adding the extra hour or two will be easy. And going from 8pm-10am is really easy since you're asleep for most of it anyway (especially if you're following the bedtime routine habit).

Most of these habits compliment each other, so fasting will help you sleep better...
> Better sleep will help reduce food cravings
> Fewer food cravings make fasting easier
> Better sleep and less food digesting will make you feel more energetic
> More energy will make training easier and more productive
> When your training is going well, you'll be more inclined to eat better too and avoid junk food...

It's easy to see how these habits compliment each other and promote good health. You can also see how most "Diets" are completely unnecessary and even damaging, when all you need to do is understand how small changes and healthy habits can eliminate the need for all of the stress around diet and exercise.

Training & Exercise

This is probably the habit you'll be most unsure about - what to do, when, how much etc is all very individual so I strongly recommend getting yourself a good coach to help you establish an appropriate starting point as well as keep you progressing ad infinitum.

A good coach is worth every penny!

I also have a collection of workouts and training plans on my membership site www.MoveBetter.Club which is well worth checking out.

You'll get access to dozens of workouts ranging from 5 to 45+

minutes and using zero or minimal equipment (there are also some gym workouts too if that's your preference), and the workout library will continue to grow.

Failing that, invest some time and money into researching training protocols and see what feels like the best fit for you - there are plenty of programs online and thousands of books available.

Just be sure to take a sensible approach and if something doesn't feel right, look at how you can change it.

Again, I can't recommend enough hiring a coach to guide you - you are unique. Your abilities, fitness levels, flexibility, confidence, injuries and medical conditions, available equipment, past exercise experience, schedule, work and family time etc all play a part in setting up your training plan and it'll cost you a lot of time and effort trying to figure it out for yourself - a bit like all the years you've spent trying to figure out what "Diet" is best... there isn't one, just one that's right for you, at that time.

An Online Coach could be a good option too if you're happy to go and do the work yourself and don't want or need someone standing over you while you do so. You can go to www.MoveBetter.Club and check out the "Work with Mark" section if you'd like to work with me.

There's no perfect program, just some things to bear in mind and try to cover in your program.

Predominantly, that you *need* to include strength work (functional training, not bodybuilding style workouts), as well as "cardio" (at a range of different intensities and each in varying amounts), mobility work and recovery.

This may well be my next book, but until then, find something you enjoy and will actually *want* to do, and then add in any aspects of fitness that it doesn't cover.

Again, check out www.MoveBetter.Club to get access to *my* content.

THANKYOU!

I'd just like to say Thank You for reading this book!

I really hope it helps you gain better control over your habits and lifestyle and I *know* it can make a HUGE difference to your life.

The key to success with health and fitness is to create healthy habits and eliminate bad habits.

Once something becomes a part of your lifestyle, without the need to think about it, it becomes effortless, and these 9 habits really do underlie everything else and create a solid foundation for lifelong health.

Please let me know what you think of the book, all feedback is welcome.

What did you like most?
What did you like least?
Is there anything missing you'd like me to include?
Is anything unclear?

And finally, *please* do let me know how you get on with these habits - I want to hear all of your successes!

Weight/Fat loss... Better health markers... More energy... More confidence... Less stress... Any reductions in medications... ANYTHING you think this has helped you with.

You can tag me or contact me through social media or via email.
YouTube - @Move-Better
Instagram - @MoveBetterClub

Twitter - @MoveBetterClub
Facebook - MoveBetterClubOnline
E-mail - Mark@MoveBetter.Club

BONUSES/RESOURCES

For the resources mentioned in this book, please visit www.MoveBetter.Club/NoDiet where you'll find all the resources mentioned and more...